HEALTHY CHOICE

50 delicious creative vegetable salads

Henry White

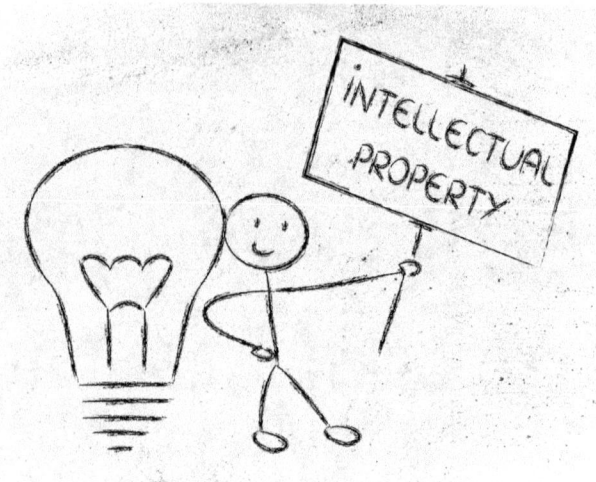

Table of Contents

Introduction

Our health is dependent on our diet. Think about our bodies as a machine. When you give a machine the wrong fuel or cheap, subpar fuel, your machine only will not run right or for as long as it should. Food is our fuel. Fad diets are everywhere, and there is no doubt about that. It can seem like every diet has a doctor backing it and testimonials from people just like you claiming it's the best diet out there. You might have tried some of these diets, but you were displeased with the results.

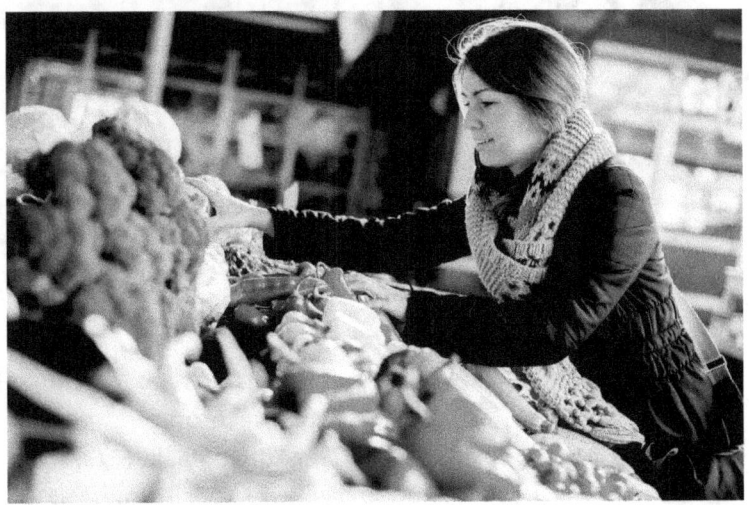

Why vegetable salads?

Gone are the days when vegetable salads were described as just tomatoes and lettuce. Thanks to the few food enthusiasts and chefs who embraced the vegetable salads that not only probe our food hankering but also trigger our rational fib of healthy living.

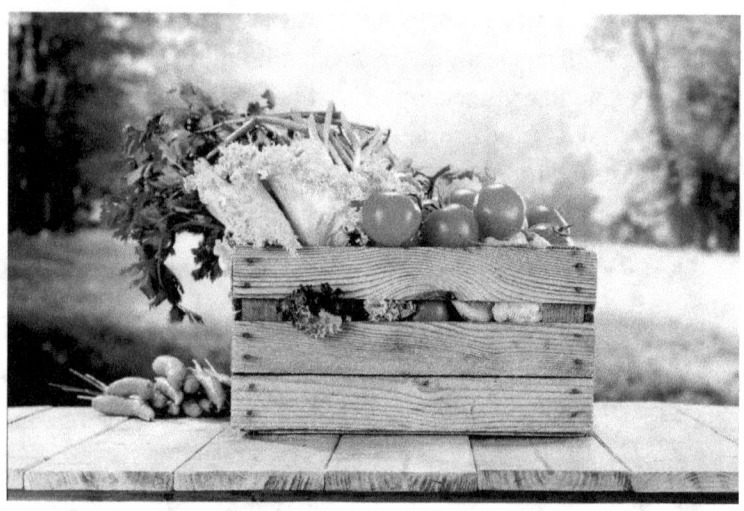

These vegetables include kale, spinach, peppers, Arugula, cabbage, Bok Choy, collard greens, Broccoli, Brussels sprouts, Celery, etc. This list also incorporates botanical fruits like pumpkins. This Vegetable Salad Cookbook contains 50 healthy and delicious salad recipes. It also provides all the relevant knowledge needed to understand this popular lifestyle choice.

Mexican salad

(Ready in 15 minutes. 2 servings)

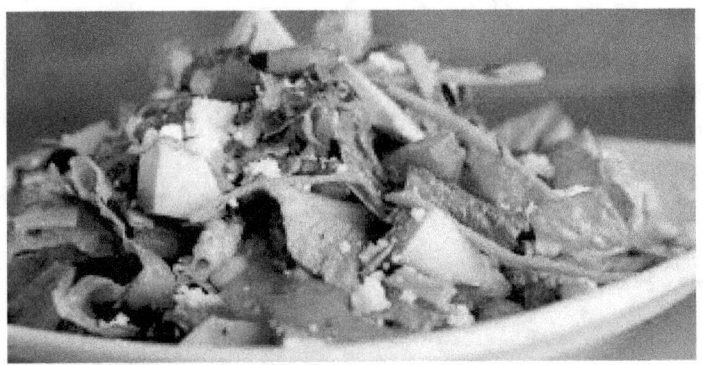

Ingredients
- ✓ 400g cooed red beans 400g cooked
- ✓ 100g round tomatoes
- ✓ 1 ripe avocado
- ✓ 2 fennel leaves
- ✓ 1 small onion
- ✓ 2 c. in lime soup
- ✓ 1 c. tablespoons olive oil
- ✓ 1 chili paste tip
- ✓ 1 c. chopped fresh coriander
- ✓ Salt
- ✓ pepper

Instructions
1. Cut two tomatoes into quarters, avocados intocubes, and fennel into thin strips.
2. Mixer roughly the third tomato, onion, lime juice, olive oil, chili paste and cilantro.
3. Add salt and pepper sauce. Mix all ingredients and serve with corn tortilla.

Sweet and sour salad

(Ready in 10 minutes. 2 servings)

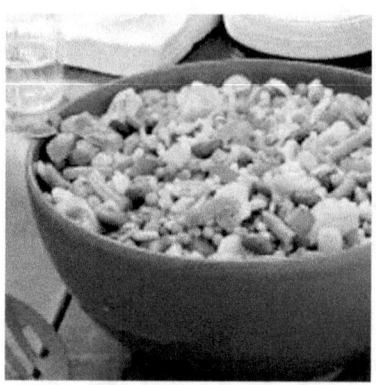

Ingredients:
- ✓ 2 tablespoons olive oil,
- ✓ 1 grapefruit diced,
- ✓ 1/2 mango diced,
- ✓ 1/2 teaspoon sesame seeds,
- ✓ 3 cups lettuce, sliced
- ✓ 1/2 avocado,
- ✓ Salt and pepper.

Preparation

1. In a bowl, mix the grapefruit, mango and sesame seeds with oil.
2. Then add the lettuce and avocado. Season and taste.

Vegetable salad

(Ready in 10 minutes. 2 servings)

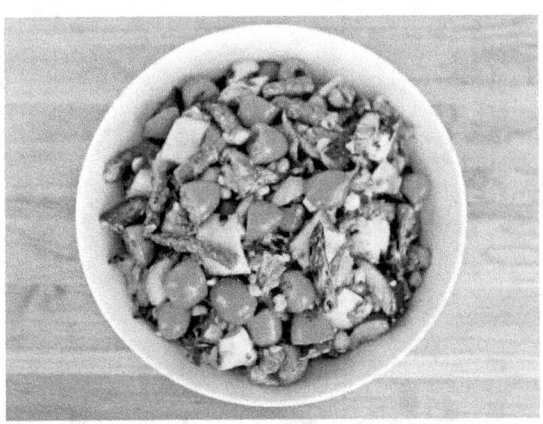

Ingredients:
- ✓ *2 zucchini, thinly sliced,*
- ✓ *1 cup halved cherry tomatoes,*
- ✓ *1 tablespoon lemon juice,*
- ✓ *3 tablespoons balsamic vinegar*
- ✓ *1 clove garlic, minced*
- ✓ *1/2 cup chopped basil,*
- ✓ *2 tablespoon of olive oil,*
- ✓ *10 small mozzarella balls cut in half,*
- ✓ *Salt and pepper.*

Preparation

1. *Place all your ingredients in your dish, add dressing and mix well.*
2. *Season and you can taste this delicious summer salad!*

Beet salad

(Ready in 5 minutes. 2 servings)

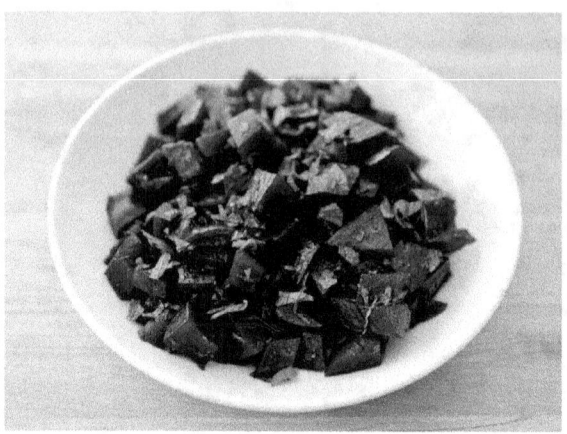

Ingredients:
- ✓ 100 g feta, ,
- ✓ Fresh basil,
- ✓ 3 cooked beets,
- ✓ 1 tablespoon of nuts,
- ✓ 1Tablespoon vinegar,
- ✓ Salt and pepper.

Preparation

1. Wash and dry your mash.
2. Cut your beets and feta your dice. Place your ingredients in a bowl.
3. Add the chopped basil and dressing. You just have to mix and enjoy your salad!

Pasta salad

(Ready in 5 minutes. 2 servings)

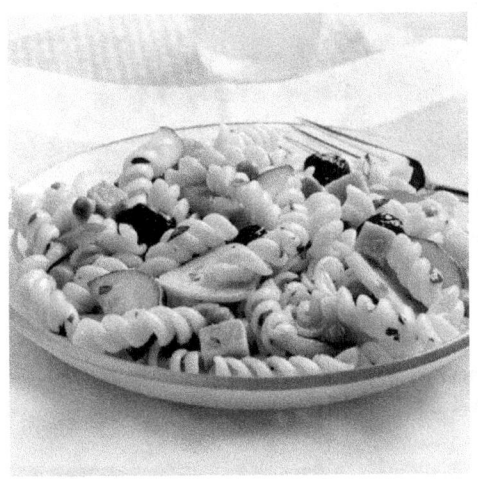

Ingredients:

- ✓ Pasta,
- ✓ 2 avocados,
- ✓ 1/4 cup basil leaves,
- ✓ 1/4 cup grated Parmesan cheese,
- ✓ 1 tablespoon of olive oil,
- ✓ 2 tomatoes,
- ✓ 1/2 red onion
- ✓ 2 tablespoons of lemon juice,
- ✓ Salt
- ✓ Pepper.

Preparation
1. Cook your pasta according to package directions. In your dish, mix the pasta, ham, avocado, tomatoes, onion and basil.
2. Add the parmesan, olive oil, lemon juice, salt and pepper.

Salad greque

(Ready in 5 minutes. 2 servings)

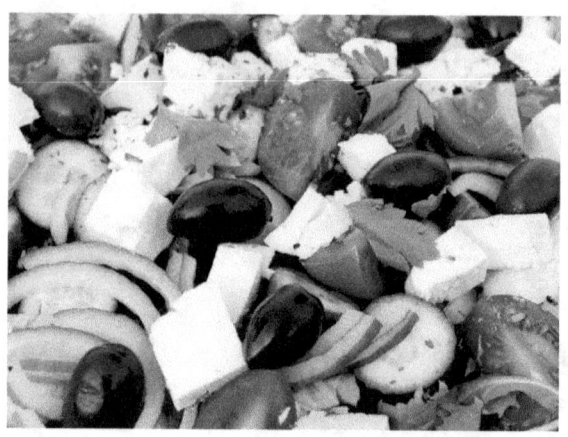

Ingredients:
- ✓ 5 cups chopped lettuce,
- ✓ 1 small red onion, thinly sliced,
- ✓ 1 cucumber, thinly sliced,
- ✓ 1/2 cup cherry tomatoes, halved
- ✓ 1/4 cup olives, goat cheese
- ✓ 1/4 cup crumbled,
- ✓ Salt and pepper.

Preparation
1. Place all your ingredients in your dish, pour vinaigrette, salt and pepper and you can taste.

Asian salad

(Ready in 10 minutes. 4 servings)

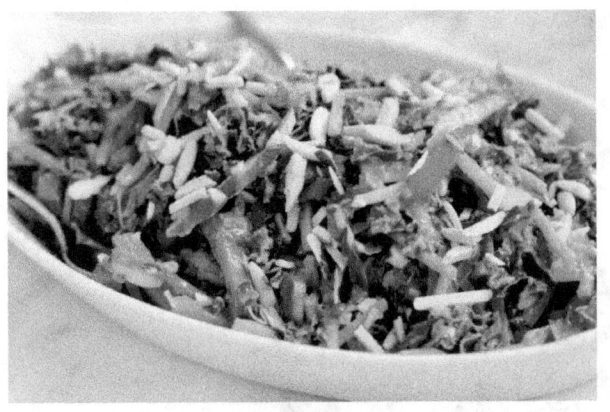

Ingredients:
- ✓ 1 cup white rice,
- ✓ 12 broccoli florets,
- ✓ 1 tablespoon of olive oil,
- ✓ 70 g of sliced chicken,
- ✓ Salt,
- ✓ Pepper,
- ✓ 1 green onion, thinly sliced,
- ✓ Soy sauce,
- ✓ 1/2 cup of chicken broth,
- ✓ Lemon juice,
- ✓ 1 tablespoon cider vinegar,
- ✓ 2 cloves minced garlic.

Preparation
2. In a large saucepan cook the rice. Then cook the broccoli to steam.
3. Heat the olive oil then add the chicken. Stir in chicken broth, soy sauce and garlic in your stove. Incorporate all your ingredients in a dish and enjoy!

Tomato, mozzarella, and basil salad

(Ready in 20 minutes. 2 servings)

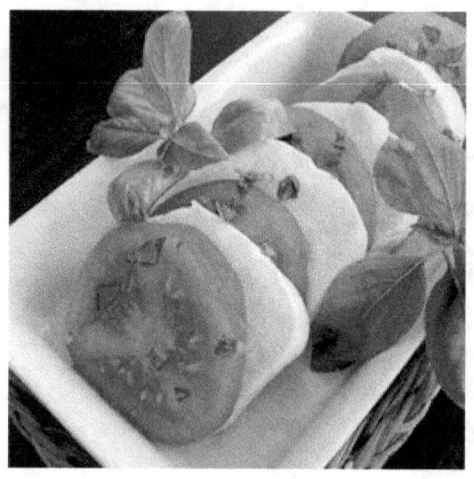

Ingredients:
- ✓ 1 loaf of bread,
- ✓ 3 tablespoons extra virgin olive oil,
- ✓ 1 bowl of cherry tomatoes,
- ✓ 8 mini mozzarella balls
- ✓ 100 g chicken,
- ✓ 1 bunch basil leaves.

Preparation
1. Preheat oven to 190 degrees. Cut your baguette in half horizontally.
2. Brush pastry with olive oil on both sides of the bread.
3. Cut your bread into small pieces and cook in oven for 10 minutes.
4. In a bowl, add the tomatoes, mozzarella, chicken cut into small pieces, basil and 1 tablespoon of olive oil. Mix with the bread and taste.

Caesar

(Ready in 5hrs. 4 servings)

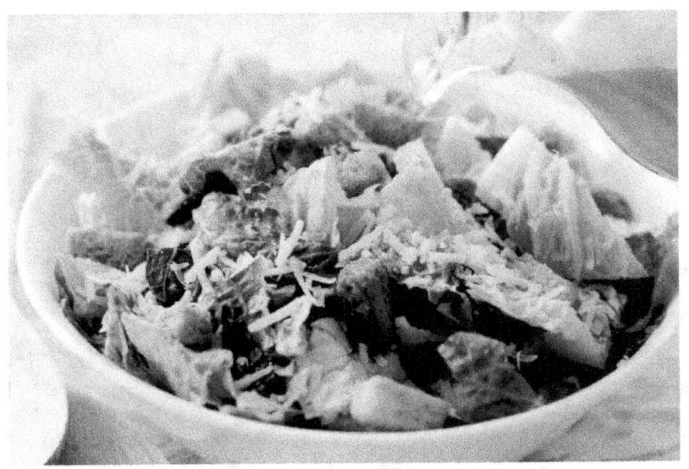

Ingredients:
- ✓ *Green salad, parmesan,*
- ✓ *4 crackers,*
- ✓ *A few croutons,*
- ✓ *1/2 lemon,*
- ✓ *1/2 shallot,*
- ✓ *Cumin or paprika,*
- ✓ *Salt,*
- ✓ *Pepper.*

Preparation
1. *Cut to pieces 2 rusks and then add your spices, salt and pepper.*
2. *Mix with your white breadcrumbs and bake 10 minutes at the stove.*
3. *Rub 2 toasts with garlic and mix all your ingredients in a bowl, add the dressing and you can taste.*

Thai salad

(Ready in 10 minutes. 2 servings)

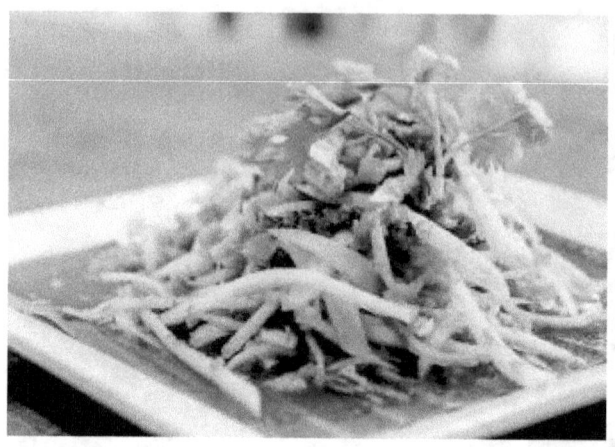

Ingredients:
- ✓ 2 cucumbers,
- ✓ 2 mangoes,
- ✓ 1 red pepper,
- ✓ 2 tablespoons peanuts,
- ✓ Coriander 6 rods,
- ✓ 2 tablespoons sherry,
- ✓ 5 tablespoons of peanut oil,
- ✓ Salt and pepper.

Preparation
1. Cut your cucumber into thin slices.
2. Peel and cut the mango into small cubes and finely chop the peppers and chop the coriander.
3. Add all your ingredients in a bowl and stir in your dressing and season.

Cucumber tagliatelle

(Ready in 10 minutes. 2 servings)

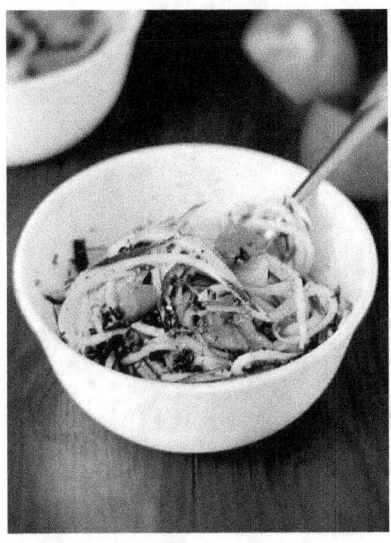

Ingredients:
- ✓ 1 zucchini,
- ✓ 1 small yellow squash,
- ✓ 1 ear of corn,
- ✓ Goat cheese,
- ✓ Basil,
- ✓ Red pepper flakes,
- ✓ Salt and pepper.

Preparation
1. Peel zucchini and squash lengthwise.
2. Place your preparation in a bowl and add corn kernels and 2 tablespoons of dressing.
3. Then add salt, pepper mill and then the goat cheese and basil.

Quinoa salad

(Ready in 10 minutes. 2 servings)

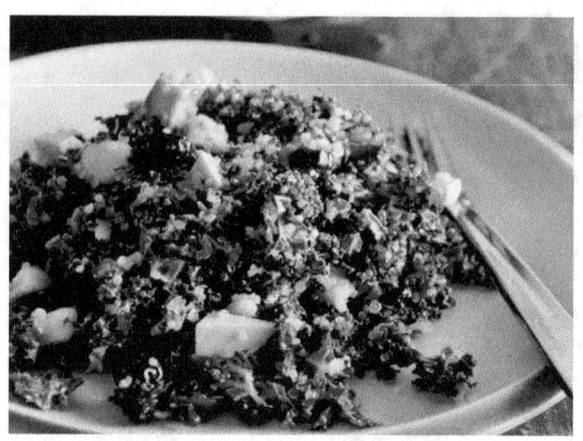

Ingredients:
- ✓ *1 cup quinoa,*
- ✓ *2 cucumbers,*
- ✓ *1 small red onion, diced,*
- ✓ *1 tomato,*
- ✓ *1 bunch parsley,*
- ✓ *2 bunches of mint leaves,*
- ✓ *2 tablespoons olive oil,*
- ✓ *1 / 4 cup red wine vinegar,*
- ✓ *1 lemon,*
- ✓ *1 teaspoon salt,*
- ✓ *2 teaspoons pepper*
- ✓ *1 diced avocado.*

Preparation
1. *Cook the quinoa and stir well. Transfer it to a bowl and add the cucumber, onion, tomato, vinegar, lemon juice, parsley, mint, olive oil, salt and pepper and mix well.*
2. *Add the avocado and serve.*

Blueberry salad

(Ready in 5minutes. 2 servings)

Ingredients:
- ✓ *6 cups of spinach,*
- ✓ *1 cup blueberries,*
- ✓ *1 chopped mango,*
- ✓ *1/2 red onion,*
- ✓ *1/2 cucumber,*
- ✓ *1 cup nuts.*
- ✓ *For the dressing:*
- ✓ *1 cup basil leaves,*
- ✓ *1 clove garlic,*
- ✓ *3 tablespoons honey,*
- ✓ *1/2 teaspoon pepper,*
- ✓ *1/2 teaspoon coarse salt,*
- ✓ *1/2 cup vinegar apple cider,*
- ✓ *2 tablespoons of olive oil.*

Preparation
1. *Wash your ingredients and place them into your dish.*
2. *Place the dressing ingredients in a blender and mix.*
3. *Serve over your salad.*

Fruit-mix salad

(Ready in 5 minutes. 2 servings)

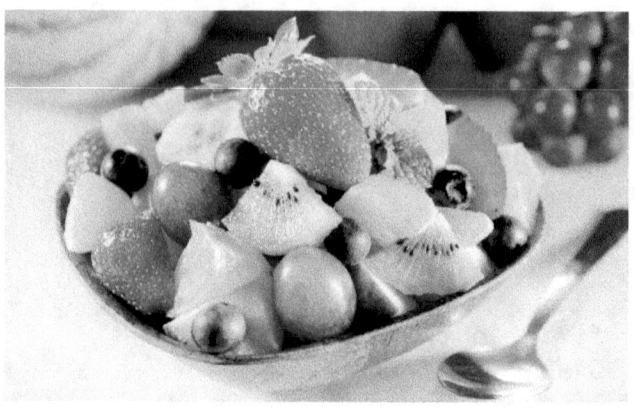

Ingredients:
- ✓ *1 pineapple,*
- ✓ *2 kiwis,*
- ✓ *12 strawberries,*
- ✓ *½ melon*
- ✓ *1/4 watermelon,*
- ✓ *1 lime,*
- ✓ *2 tablespoons maple syrup*
- ✓ *1 cup blackberries*
- ✓ *1 pinch cayenne pepper.*

Preparation
1. *In a bowl, pour the lemon juice, add the maple syrup and cayenne pepper.*
2. *Peel and slice all your fruit and* place them in a bowl.
3. Pour your juice to accompany.

Summer salad with buckwheat, apricots, almonds, arugula and fennel

(Ready in 3minutes. 4 servings)

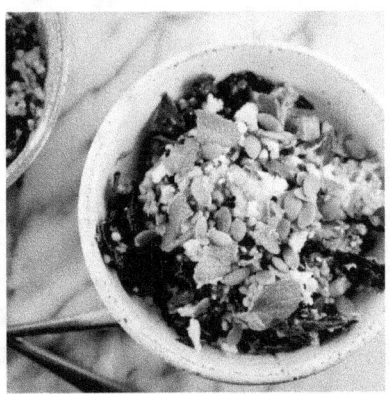

Ingredients
- ✓ 400 g of buckwheat
- ✓ 4 fresh and ripe apricots
- ✓ Half fennel, thinly sliced
- ✓ A rocket handle
- ✓ A handful (about 75g) of almonds
- ✓ 10 g fresh basil, chopped

For the sauce:
- ✓ 3 tbsp. olive oil
- ✓ 1 tbsp. vinegar
- ✓ 1 tbsp. almond purée
- ✓ 1/2 tbsp. mustard "old"
- ✓ a fresh sprig of basil
- ✓ salt + pepper

Preparation
1. Square basil rod in olive oil for a few hours.
2. Cook the buckwheat.
3. Cut apricots into thin strips (finer than mine!)
4. Put the salad ingredients in a bowl.
5. Mix the sauce ingredients (without the basil sprig) and pour over salad.

Quinoa salad, carrots and arugula

(Ready in 10 minutes. 2 servings)

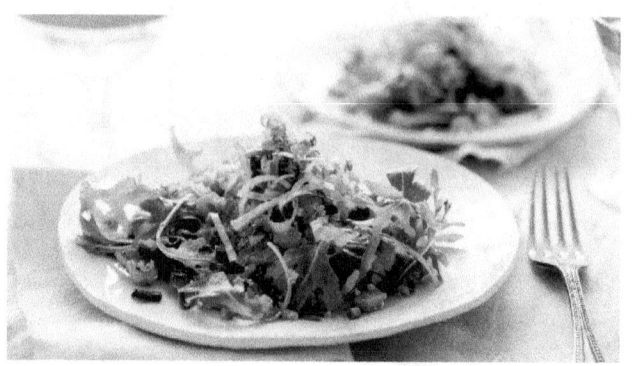

Ingredients
- ✓ 2 glasses of quinoa –
- ✓ 1 carrot
- ✓ 1 small handful of arugula (about 15g)
- ✓ Juice of half a lemon
- ✓ 1 to 2 tablespoons of olive oil (to taste)
- ✓ Salt

Preparation
Rinse quinoa and cook it in salted water.
1. Wash and peel the carrots. Cut into small dice. Wash the rocket and expand it finely. Squeeze the lemon and reserve juice.
2. Place the cooked and drained quinoa in a bowl. Add the carrots, arugula, olive oil and half the lemon juice. Mix well and add salt as needed. Enjoy warm as cold.

Grated parsnip salad with hazelnuts

(Ready in 20minutes. 2 servings)

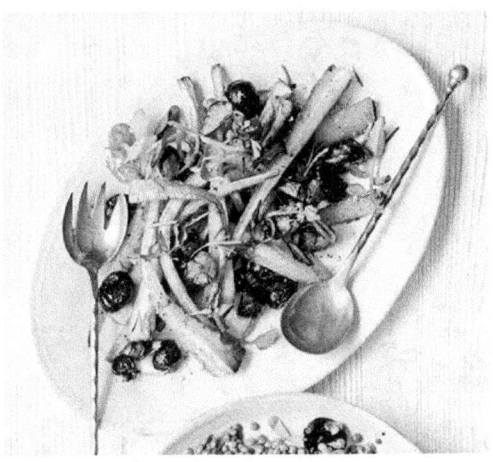

Ingredients
- ✓ 4 small parsnips
- ✓ 30 g Parmesan
- ✓ 40 g hazelnuts
- ✓ 3 tablespoons of hazelnut oil
- ✓ 1 tbsp cider vinegar
- ✓ 1 tsp mustard
- ✓ Salt and pepper

Preparation
1. Peel the parsnips and grate them
2. Mix in a bowl the vinegar, mustard, and hazelnut oil. Salt and pepper.
3. Coarsely chop the hazelnuts.
4. Arrange on plates grated parsnips, hazelnuts, and parmesan shavings.
5. Pour the vinaigrette and pepper again.

Raw pumpkin salad

(Ready in 20 minutes. 4 servings)

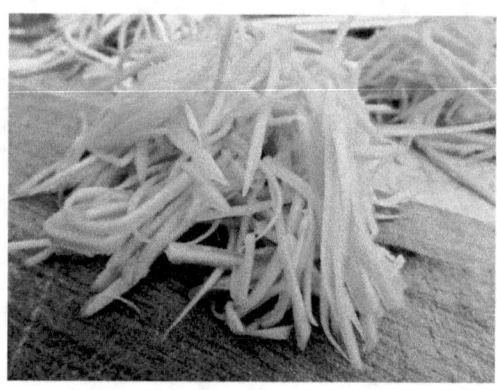

Ingredients
- ✓ *1 medium pumpkin, about 20 cm in diameter*
- ✓ *1 c. c. clean ground cumin*
- ✓ *1 c. c. clean turmeric*
- ✓ *1 c. c. scoop of ground nutmeg*
- ✓ *Olive oil, salt*
- ✓ *50g almonds*
- ✓ *50g shelled walnuts*
- ✓ *1 handful parsley / fresh chives OR 1 handful of raisins*

Preparation
1. *Preheat oven to 160 ° C to slightly toast the nuts for 10 minutes.*
2. *Coarsely chop nuts and almonds.*
3. *Peel the pumpkin, remove the seeds, and grate.*
4. *In a large bowl put the pumpkin, walnuts, almonds. Sprinkle over the spices, salt and add a good slug of olive oil (about 3-4 Tbsp. S.).*
5. *Add parsley then either / finely chopped chives or raisins.*
6. *Mix well, taste for grinding salt and spices to taste.*

Raw pepper salad with sunflower seeds.
(Ready in 15 minutes. 3 servings)

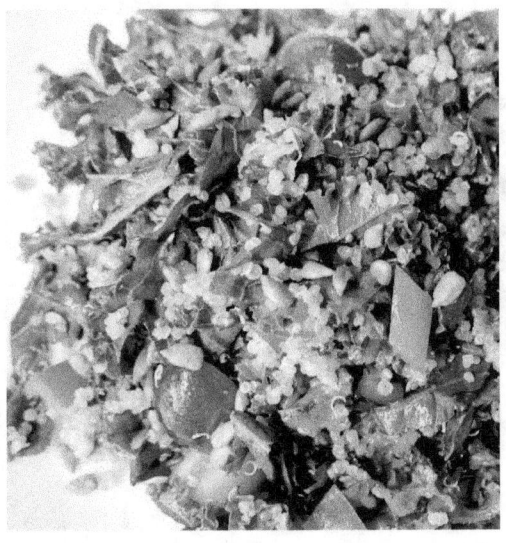

Ingredients
- ✓ 1 red pepper
- ✓ 100 g rice
- ✓ 2-3 tbsp. sunflower
- ✓ 3 tbsps. vinaigrette
- ✓ 1 bowlof black olives

Preparation
1. Wash and cut a fine red pepper into very small pieces. Meanwhile, cook rice
2. After cooking and cooling rice, add to salad of peppers and olives
3. Mix together and add sunflower seeds
4. Season with a vinaigrette or make available a base oil, vinegar, salt, pepper.

Red cabbage with green aniseed
(Ready in 15minutes. 2 servings)

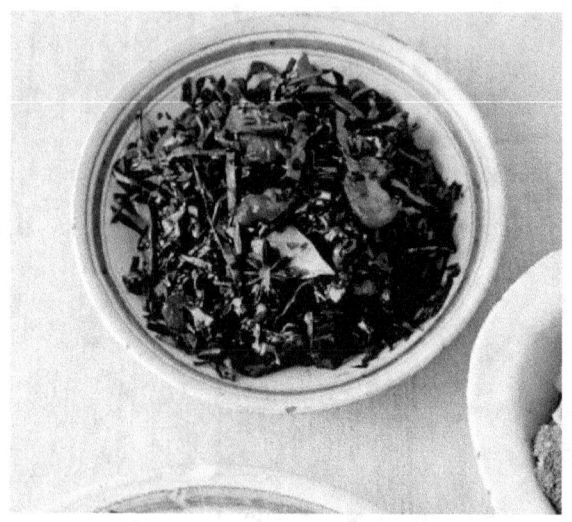

Ingredients (serves 6):
- ✓ 1/2 red cabbage
- ✓ 4 tablespoons of balsamic vinegar
- ✓ 1 tablespoon of grains of aniseed green
- ✓ 4 tablespoons of raisins

Preparation
1. Slice the red cabbage. Add dressing, green anise seeds and currants.
2. Mix.
3. marinate before serving

The real Lebanese tabbouleh

(Ready in 25minutes. 4 servings)

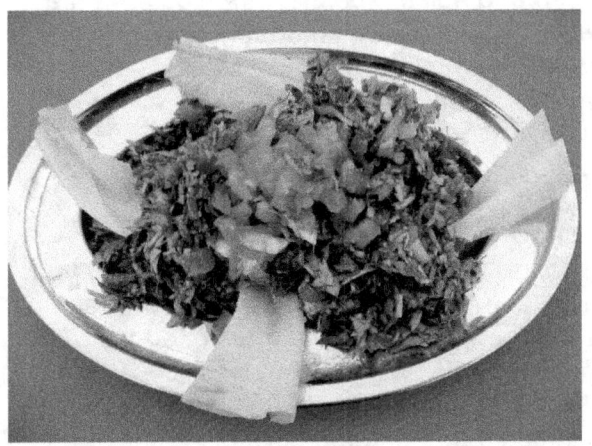

Ingredients (for 5 people):-
- ✓ *4 large tomatoes farms*
- ✓ *1bunch of onions green*
- ✓ *2 boots Parsley FLAT*
- ✓ *1 bunch mint fresh*
- ✓ *1 small handful of medium brown bulgur (cracked wheat)*
- ✓ *1 lemon*
- ✓ *3 tablespoons of olive oil*
- ✓ *2 pinches of salt*

Preparation
1. *Puta handful of bulgur in a bowl of water for 15 minutes and leave to soften.*
2. *Wash and hull the parsley, then cut it with a knife (or scissors if you prefer).*
3. *Repeat with mint, you must obtain approximately 1 cm leaves.*
4. *Put everything in a bowl.*
5. *Cut the green onions and the tomatoes into small cubes and put them in the bowl.*
6. *Remove bulger from water, and squeeze with hands to wring.Put it in the bowl with the rest.*
7. *Press 1 whole lemon and sprinkle the contents of the bowl. Add salt and 3 tablespoons of olive oil.*

   The appearance of tabbouleh should be bright, to indicate that enough olive oil.

Mishmash of melon, mozzarella, and avocado

(Ready in 20 minutes. 4 servings)

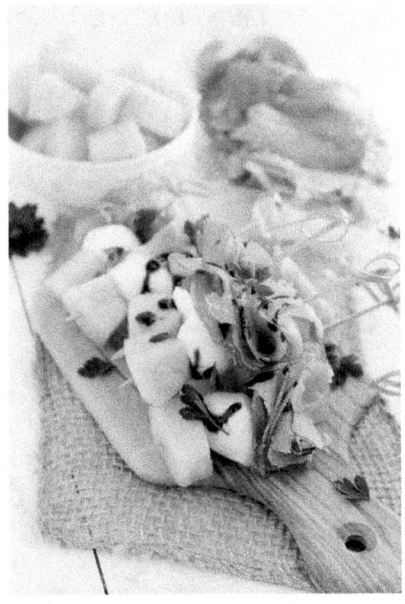

Ingredients
- ✓ *1 melon ripe*
- ✓ *1 avocado*
- ✓ *mozzarella (purchased in small balls)*
- ✓ *black olives*
- ✓ *cherry tomatoes (optional)*
- ✓ *seeds sesame*
  For the sauce:
  - *a lemon*
  - *6 tablespoons olive oil*
  - *salt and pepper*
  - *herbs: dill , chives , parsley dish, chervil ...*

Preparation
1. *Prepare small individual plates.*
2. *Form balls with a melon baller with melon and avocado.*
3. *Arrange nicely on plates with mozzarella balls.*
4. *Sprinkle with black olives, pitted and cut into thin strips.*
5. *Season by premixing the ingredients for the sauce.*
6. *Sprinkle with sesame seeds.*

Calamari salad

(Ready in 1 hour 45minutes. 6 servings)

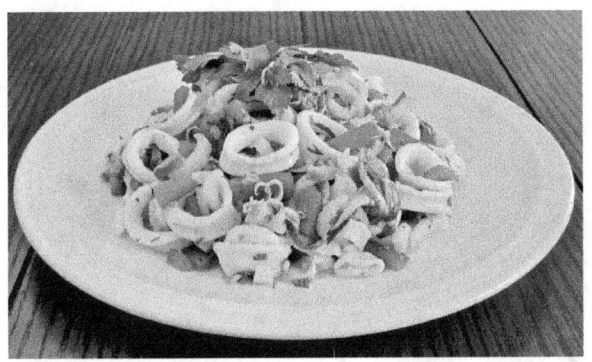

Ingredients (serves 6):
- ✓ 600 g squid
- ✓ balsamic vinegar
- ✓ 1/4 cup grape dry
- ✓ olive oil
- ✓ onion minced red
- ✓ 1 cup dry white wine
- ✓ 4 tomatoes peeled, seeded and chopped
- ✓ 1 / 4 cup parsley chopped
- ✓ nuts, to taste
- ✓ 1 pinch of paprika and chili powder

Preparation
1. Soak the raisins in 2 tablespoons balsamic vinegar for 30 minutes and drain.
2. Cut the squid bodies into pieces of about 5 x 5 cm and put them in a baking dish. Add a little olive oil, wine, and tomatoes and cook 1 hour in the oven, covered.
3. When pricking the flesh with the tip of a knife it has no resistance, it's cooked!
4. Stir parsley, raisins, paprika, chili and pine nuts. Add salt and pepper, add 1 tablespoon of balsamic vinegar (or more according to your taste).

Avocado lime

(Ready in 10minutes. 4 servings)

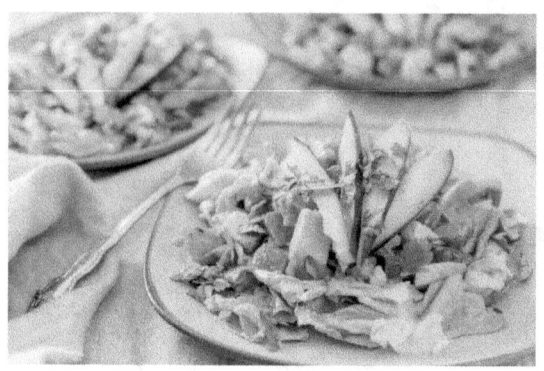

Ingredients

- ✓ 2 avocados
- ✓ 8 lettuce leaves
- ✓ sorbet lemon
- ✓ oil
- ✓ balsamic vinegar
- ✓ salt , pepper

Preparation

1. Wash the lettuce leaves, drain and set aside.
2. Peel the avocados, cut into 8 slices and drizzle with lemon juice net to prevent them from darkening. Book.
3. Make vinaigrette lightly with 1 tablespoon of vinegar, 2 tablespoons of oil, a pinch of salt and a pinch of pepper.
4. In each plate, place 2 lettuce leaves coarsely chopped, drizzle with dressing, have over 4 slices of avocado, add a scoop of sorbet with lime in the center. Serve immediately.

Grated carrot salad with almonds and tuna

(Ready in 10minutes. 4 servings)

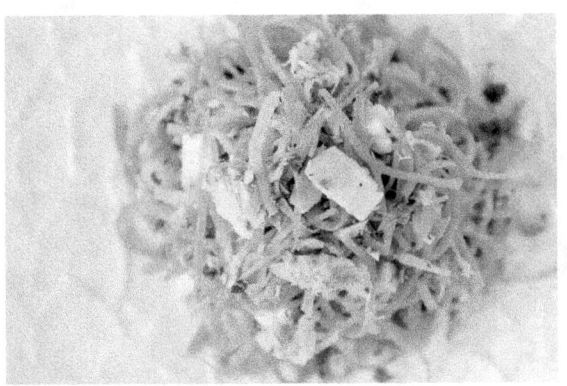

Ingredients
- ✓ *5 large carrots1 can of tuna*
- ✓ *1 lemon*
- ✓ *150 g whole almonds*
- ✓ *2 tablespoons cilantro chopped*
- ✓ *2 cloves garlic*
- ✓ *salt , pepper*
- ✓ *olive oil*

Preparation:
1. *Grate carrots, add the tuna, almonds, coriander and finely chopped garlic, a little olive oil, salt, and pepper.*

(Ready in 10 minutes. 4 servings)

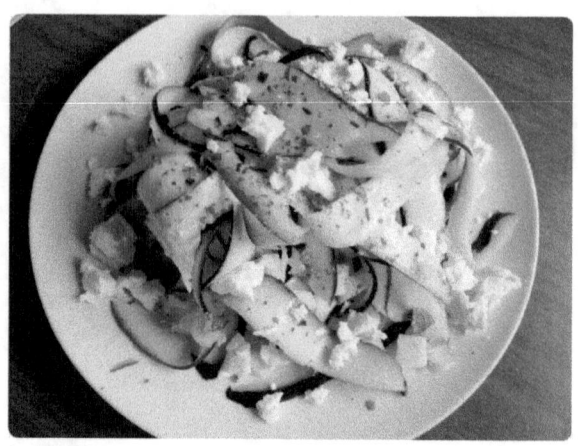

Ingredients

- ✓ 2 large zucchini
- ✓ 200g feta (oil)
- ✓ 2 large onions
- ✓ 4 tomatoes
- ✓ black olives
- ✓ basil
- ✓ salt , pepper

Preparation

2. *Cut zucchini into thin slices, and make them disgorge with coarse salt in a colander about 30 minutes (until tender).*
3. *Meanwhile, cut the feta into small cubes, chop the tomatoes into small wedges, cut the onions into small pieces and blanch in salted water 2 minutes.*
4. *Put the zucchini with feta cheese, tomatoes, onions, olives in a bowl, add the basil.*
5. *Mix with a vinaigrette house (oil olive + + wine vinegar mustard).*

Fennel salad with orange

(Ready in 10 minutes. 4 servings)

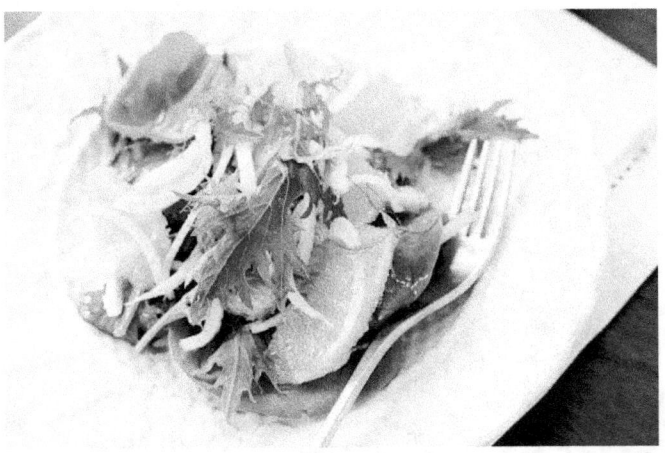

Ingredients
- ✓ 2 fennel
- ✓ 1 orange
- ✓ dill
- ✓ 5 cl of vinegar cider
- ✓ 5 cl of olive oil
- ✓ 1 tsp mustard

Preparation
1. Clean the fennel, remove the green parts and chop finely in a bowl.
2. Prepare the vinaigrette with apple cider vinegar, mustard, orange juice, salt, and pepper.
3. Sprinkle with fennel and sprinkle with chopped dill.

Salad tomatoes and kiwis Lili

(Ready in 5 minutes. 2 servings)

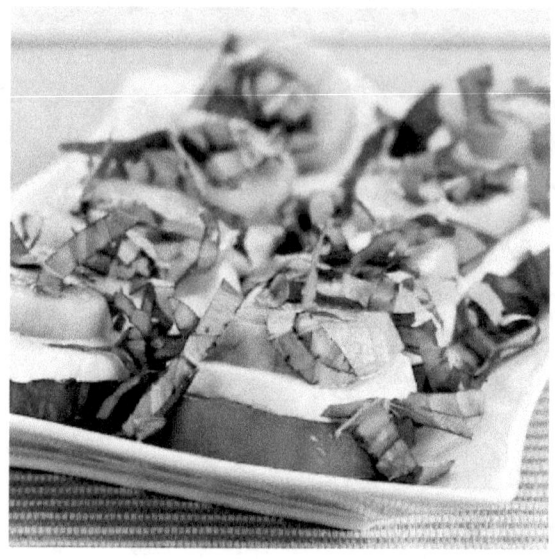

Ingredients
- ✓ 2 kiwis
- ✓ 2 tomatoes
- ✓ salt , pepper
- ✓ Oil choice
- ✓ lemon or vinegar

Preparation
1. *Peel the kiwis and tomatoes, cut into slices.*
2. *Arrange in a dish, season with salt and drizzle with a little oil, add the juice of half a lemon or a little vinegar to your preferences*

Rocket salad with parmesan and pine nuts

(Ready in 10 minutes. 4 servings)

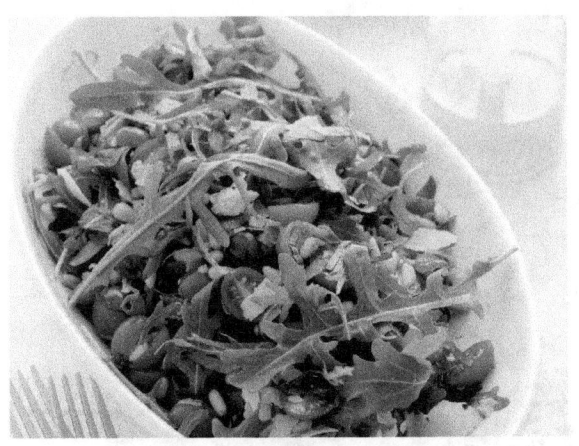

Ingredients (serves 4):
- ✓ *300 g rocket*
- ✓ *1 piece of parmesan 50g*
- ✓ *Pinions or nuts at will*

Preparation
1. *Clean the rocket. Add in a bowl of parmesan slices (easy to do with a peeler). Put pine nuts or walnuts.*
2. *Drizzle with a dressing classic made with balsamic vinegar.*
3. *In summer you can add slices of melon is delicious.*

Watermelon and feta salad

(Ready in 15 minutes. 4 servings)

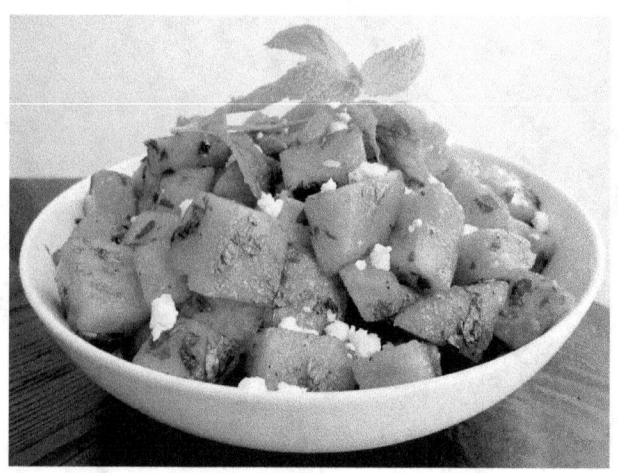

Ingredients

- ✓ *2 kg of watermelon*
- ✓ *100g feta*
- ✓ *1 tablespoon mint chopped fresh*
- ✓ *100 g black olives (Nice)*
- ✓ *1 tablespoon olive oil*

Preparation

1. *Cut the watermelon into cubes, add the feta that is also cup diced, small black olives, and sprinkle with fresh mint and drizzle with olive oil.*
2. *Mix gently, chill.*

Quinoa salad

(Ready in 30 minutes. 4 servings)

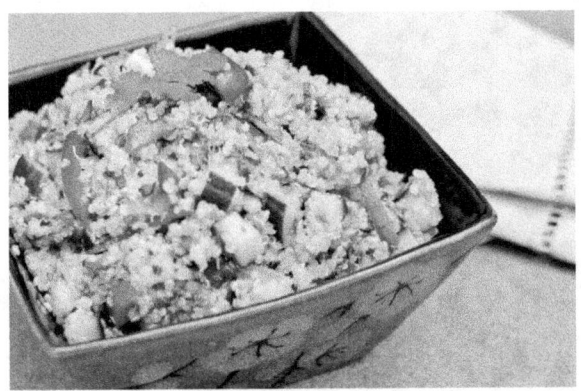

Ingredients

- ✓ 1 glass of quinoa
- ✓ 1/2 cucumber
- ✓ 2 tomatoes
- ✓ 20 sheets of mint
- ✓ 1 shallot
- ✓ olive oil
- ✓ lemon juice
- ✓ salt

Preparation:

1. Cook the quinoa for 15 minutes in boiling water. Once cooked, cool it by rinsing with cold water and let it drain in a colander.
2. While the cooked quinoa, rinse the tomatoes, remove the seeds and the juice flows out and cut tomatoes into small cubes.
3. Peel the cucumber half, remove seeds and cut it, too, into small dice. Cut finely mint and shallots.
4. Mix all the vegetables with cold quinoa. Season with lemon juice, salt and olive oil!

Spicy potato salad

(Ready in 30 minutes. 4 servings)

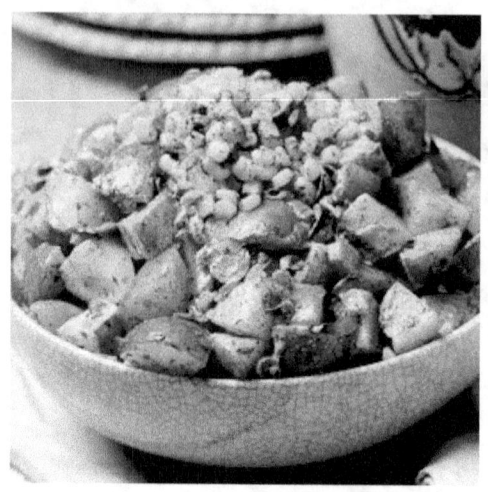

Ingredients

- ✓ 500 g of potatoes
- ✓ 3 tablespoons olive oil
- ✓ Juice of 1/2 lemon
- ✓ 3 tablespoons of seeds sesame
- ✓ 1 tablespoon coffee paprika
- ✓ 1 teaspoon cumin
- ✓ 1 tablespoon coffee coriander ground
- ✓ salt and pepper

Preparation

1. Peel, cut potatoes into small cubes and boil.
2. Mix all the spices with olive oil and lemon juice and pour the potatoes. Stir well and leave a little rest.
3. Broil dry the sesame seeds (careful, it goes very fast!).
4. Mix the salad and serve.

Tuna and pesto pasta salad

(Ready in 27 minutes. 6 servings)

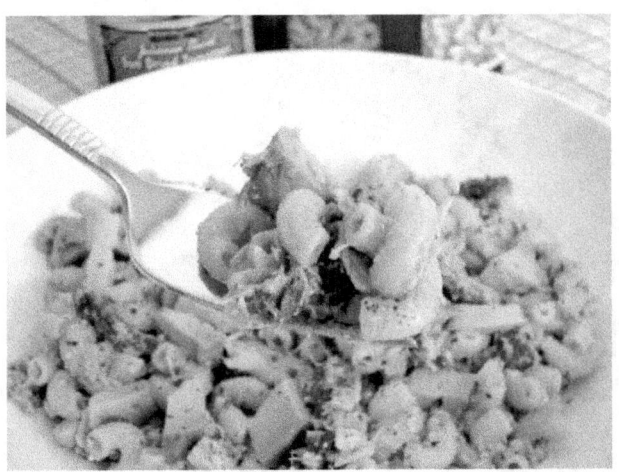

Ingredients

- ✓ 500 g of green and red pasta (with vegetables)
- ✓ 200 g of tuna
- ✓ 3 to 4 tablespoons pesto
- ✓ salt and pepper
- ✓ fresh basil

Preparation

1. While cooking the pasta in boiling salted water, mix tuna in a large bowl with pesto depending on your taste.
2. When the pasta is cooked, rinse under cold water to stop cooking and mixing with tuna mixture. Serve cold.

Tuna salad with banana
(Ready in 15 minutes. 4 servings)

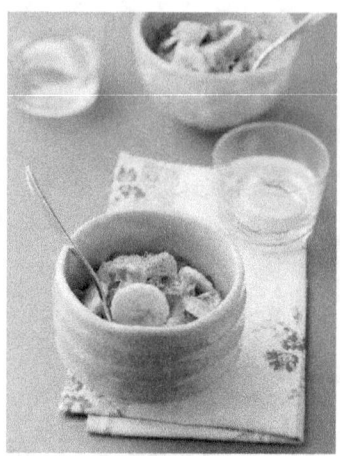

Ingredients

- ✓ *1 can of tuna Nature*
- ✓ *300 g cooked albacore tuna*
- ✓ *3 ripe barely bananas*
- ✓ *100g rice*
- ✓ *2 peppers red*
- ✓ *cream (to taste)*
- ✓ *curry (to taste)*
- ✓ *salt and pepper*
- ✓ *oil and vinegar*

Preparation

1. *Cook the rice (but beware, it must remain firm). Allow to cool.*
2. *Crumble the tuna. Cut the peppers into small cubes and bananas into slices.*
3. *Mix together and pour sauce composed of a large spoonful of cream, a pinch of salt and pepper, oil and 2 vinegar.*
4. *Sprinkle with curry.*
5. *Serve chilled.*

Tuna salad as in Mauritius.
(Ready in 5 minutes. 2 servings)

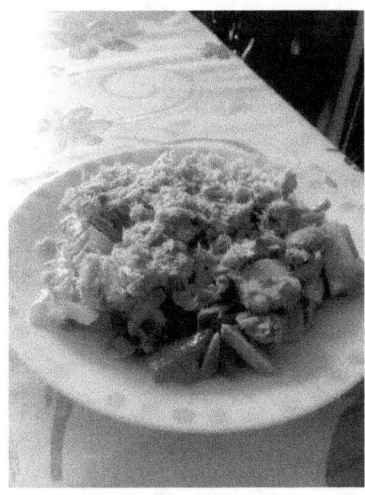

Ingredients

- ✓ 1 can of tuna in oil or water
- ✓ 1 large tomato
- ✓ 1 onion
- ✓ a few sprigs of fresh coriander
- ✓ 2 or 3 tablespoons of oil (2 tablespoons lemon juice
- ✓ salt , pepper, and green pepper if you like

Preparation

1. Peel the onion and slice as thin as possible.
2. Cut the tomato into thin slices (such as onions). Chop the coriander. Drain tuna.
3. Put all ingredients in a bowl, add salt and pepper. Let stand 10 minutes. Replace the Bluefin tuna with Albacore tuna that has the same color as the Bluefin tuna when raw.

43

Mozzarella Tomato Salad

(Ready in 10 minutes. 4 servings)

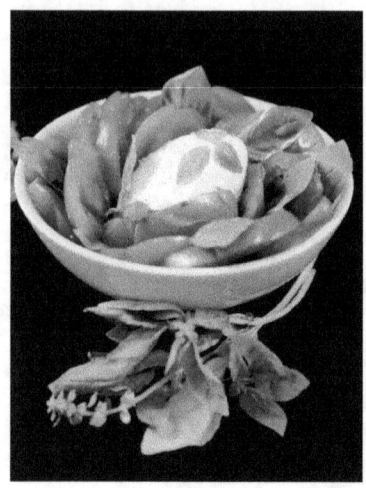

Ingredients

- ✓ *4 large tomatoes*
- ✓ *400 g of mozzarella*
- ✓ *1 bunch basil*
- ✓ *2 tablespoons balsamic vinegar*
- ✓ *5 tablespoons olive oil*
- ✓ *1 onion*
- ✓ *Salt and pepper*

Preparation
1. *Wash the basil and set aside. Cut mozzarellainto thin slices. Cut tomatoes into slices.*
2. *Peel and chop the onion.*
3. *Chop the basil and set aside.*
4. *Put in a bowl, pepper, salt, balsamic vinegar and mix; add the olive oil.*
5. *Add the mozzarella, basil and tomatoes in the bowl.*

Tomato and feta salad
(Ready in 10 minutes. 4 servings)

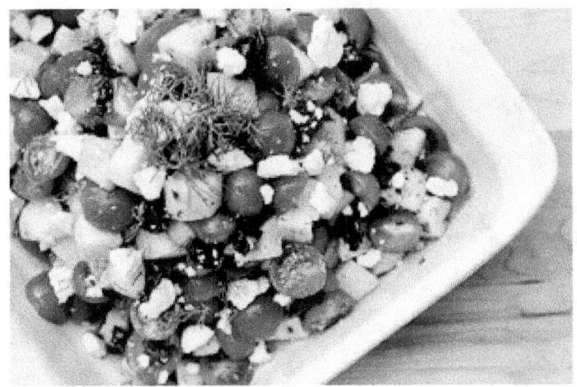

Ingredients
- ✓ *4 tomatoes cluster*
- ✓ *1 shallot*
- ✓ *200g feta*
- ✓ *pepper*
- ✓ *herbs*
- ✓ *anise*
- ✓ *olive oil*
- ✓ *1 lemon (juice)*

Preparation
1. *Cut the tomatoes in quarters.*
2. *Add coarsely chopped shallots*
3. *Cut feta into small cubes and add to the mixture.*
4. *Sprinkle with pepper, herbs and anise.*
5. *Pour olive oil and lemon juice, then mix, it's ready!*

According to taste, you can also add green or black olives.

Tomato salad with shallots

(Ready in 15 minutes. 4 servings)

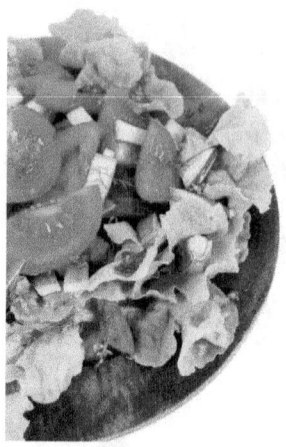

Ingredients
- ✓ 6 tomatoes market (green and red of all sizes)
- ✓ 2 shallots
- ✓ 4 tablespoons of quality olive oil
- ✓ chives fresh
- ✓ salt and pepper

Preparation
1. Cut the tomatoes into the washer over a bowl to collect the juice.
2. Slice the shallots and add to the bowl.
3. Season with olive oil, salt, pepper and finely. Chopped chives
4. Let stand, cover with a clean towel before serving (1/2 hour - 1 hour),
5. Serve with good bread for power saucer!!
6. Enjoy!

Endive salad gourmet

(Ready in 15 minutes. 4 servings)

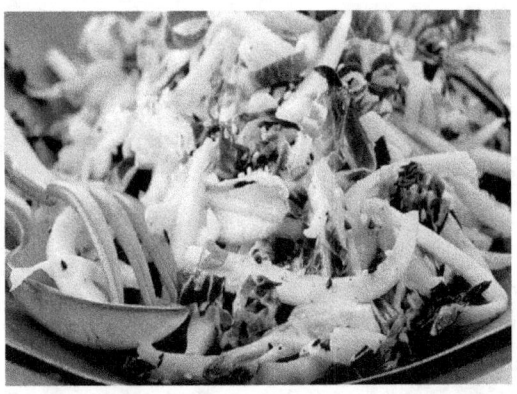

Ingredients

- ✓ *4 large endives*
- ✓ *6 slices of bacon*
- ✓ *100 g Roquefort cheese*
- ✓ *100 g county*
- ✓ *mustard*
- ✓ *vinegar cider*
- ✓ *cream*
- ✓ *pepper*

Preparation

1. *Wash and drain the endives, cut into small pieces.*
2. *Set aside in a bowl.*
3. *Add the whole endive.*
4. *Prepare a sauce with a teaspoon of mustard, 1 tablespoon vinegar 4 cider, and cream, a little pepper.*

Spinach salad with parmesan

(Ready in 10 minutes. 4 servings)

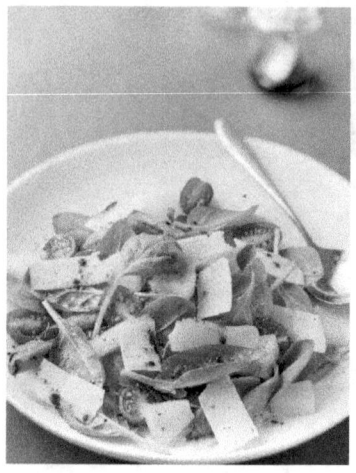

Ingredients
- ✓ *200 g young leaves of spinach*
- ✓ *10 cherry tomatoes*
- ✓ *100 g of fresh Parmesan*
- ✓ *4 slices of pineapple*
- ✓ *1 lemon*
- ✓ *2 tablespoons olive oil*
- ✓ *2 tablespoons tablespoon of rapeseed oil*
- ✓ *salt , pepper*

Preparation
1. *After choosing the most tender and clear spinach, remove stems and wash.*
2. *Prepare the sauce by mixing the salt, pepper, both oil and lemon juice. Cut the tomatoes cherries in half, add pineapple and cut spinach into small pieces*
3. *Add drained parmesan shavings, mix well and serve.*

Feta salad Grapes

(Ready in 10 minutes. 6 servings)

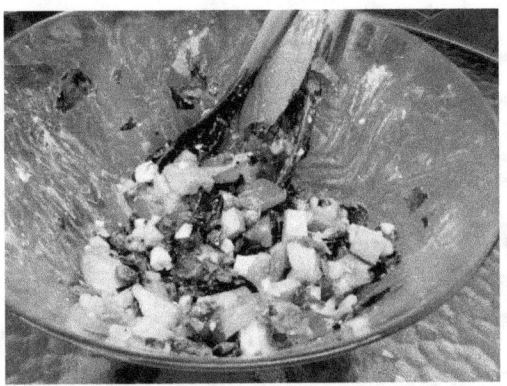

Ingredients
- ✓ 1 box corn grains
- ✓ 1 lettuce red oak leaf
- ✓ 4 small tomatoes
- ✓ 1 jar of feta cheese with herbs
- ✓ 25 g handful of grapes dry
- ✓ 2 avocados
- ✓ 5 cl vinaigrette

Preparation
1. Cut the tomatoes, avocados into small pieces. Wash the salad and prepare.
2. Put all ingredients in a large bowl.
3. Prepare the vinaigrette with oil feta jar.
4. Serve

Kale salad with cranberries and feta
(Ready in 15 minutes. 4 servings)

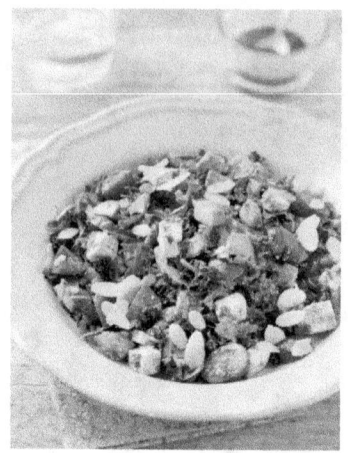

Ingredients (4 people):
- ✓ *300 g kale*
- ✓ *2 tomatoes*
- ✓ *2 avocados*
- ✓ *50 g cranberries*
- ✓ *50 g feta*
- ✓ *50g almonds*
- ✓ *1 tablespoon mustard*
- ✓ *1 tablespoon balsamic vinegar*
- ✓ *3 tablespoonsofolive oil*
- ✓ *salt*
- ✓ *pepper*

Preparation
Prepare the vinaigrette in the salad bowl: emulsify the oil with the vinegar, mustard, salt, and pepper.
Cut the kale very finely chop see. Put in the dressing.
Add the tomatoes cut into small pieces, avocados into small slices, cranberries, feta, and almonds. The salad is best when steeped in dressing for 30 minutes.

Feta salad and apples
(Ready in 10 minutes. 2 servings)

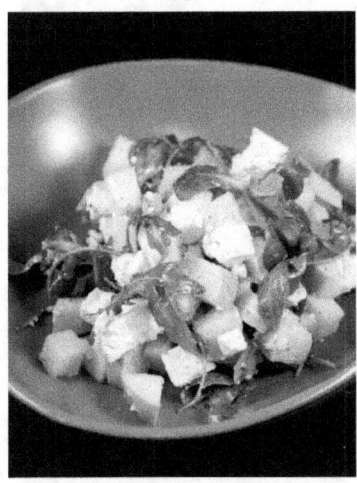

Ingredients (serves 4):
- ✓ *200 g feta kind*
- ✓ *2 apples (Granny smith)*
- ✓ *shoots of spinach*
- ✓ *for the dressing , nothing apocalyptic:*
- ✓ *mustard, vinegar, oil, salt , pepper*
- ✓ *1 teaspoon pesto*

Preparation
1. *Prepare a vinaigrette. Add the pesto*
2. *Peel the potatoes and cut into cubes.*
3. *Stir immediately to the dressing to prevent them from darkening.*
4. *Add feta cut into cubes and salad leaves. It remains for you to enjoy!*

Warm salad of peppers with cumin

(Ready in 25 minutes. 2 servings)

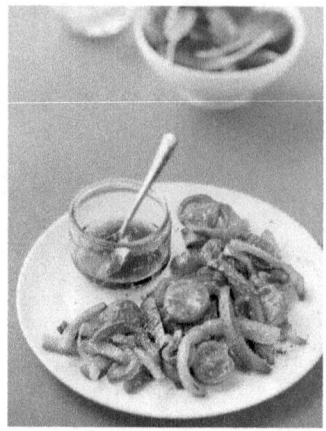

Ingredients (serves 4):
- ✓ *3 large bell peppers (1 red, 1 green and 1 yellow)*
- ✓ *4 tomatoes*
- ✓ *2 large onions purple*
- ✓ *olive oil*
- ✓ *2 tablespoons sugar powder*
- ✓ *2 tsp coffee cumin*
- ✓ *5 tablespoons wine vinegar*

Preparation
1. *Fry peppers in olive oil previously emptied of their seeds and cut into strips about 4 cm.*
2. *When the peppers begin to soften, add the sliced onions and sprinkle with sugar. When the onions are translucent, add the tomatoes into quarters and cook for five minutes, no more, otherwise they would be too soft.*
3. *Mix cumin, vinegar in a bowl and add the mixture to the vegetables. Pour into a bowl and cool to room temperature for about twenty minutes.*

Three color salad (apple, tomato, and cucumber)

(Ready in 10 minutes. 2 servings)

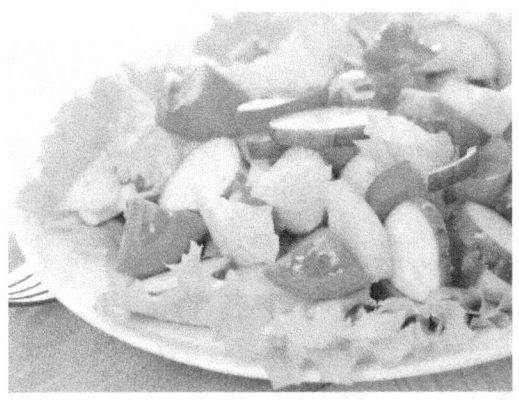

Ingredients

- ✓ *1 cucumber*
- ✓ *2 apples*
- ✓ *2 tomatoes*
- ✓ *mayonnaise*
- ✓ *sauce of soy*

Preparation

1. *Peel the cucumber and cut into very thin half-slices. Make disgorge with coarse salt.*
2. *Peel and slice the apples. Put them in the bowl with about a tablespoon of mayonnaise.*
3. *Add the tomatoes cut into small cubes.*
4. *Squeeze the cucumber ensuring that you remove the salt and put it in the bowl.*
5. *Add soy sauce net. Put in the fridge.*

Coleslaw

Ready in 30mins. 8 servings.

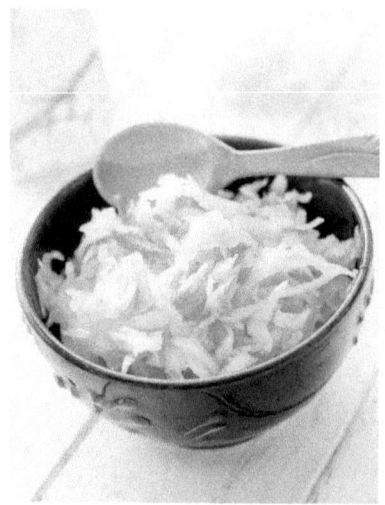

Ingredients

- ✓ 1 white cabbage
- ✓ 5 carrots
- ✓ 2 onions
- ✓ 3 tablespoons of raisins dried currant
- ✓ 3 tablespoons toasted pine nuts
- ✓ 2 tablespoons dill curved (lyophilized or branches cut finely)
- ✓ 250g mayonnaise lightened (+/- depending on individual taste, better - than +)
- ✓ salt, pepper

Preparation

1. Chop the cabbage and cucumber with the robot hand 'slicer cucumbers'
2. Grate the carrots. Chop onions by hand.
3. Make (slightly) dry roast the pine nuts in a frying pan, stirring and watching carefully.

Bobbia hot Italian salad

Ready in 1 hour. 4 servings.

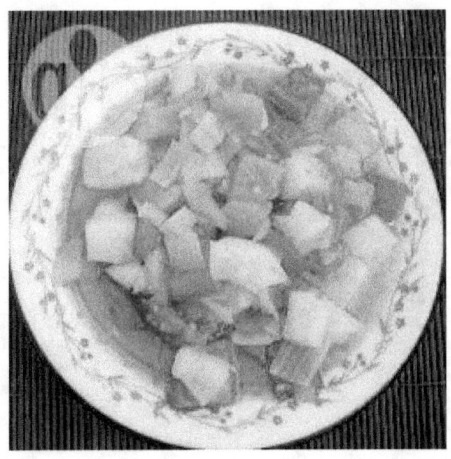

Ingredients
- ✓ *500 g large tomatoes*
- ✓ *500 g of green and red peppers, diced not too small*
- ✓ *500 g of coarsely chopped onions*
- ✓ *500g potatoes, washed and diced*
- ✓ *Salt and pepper*
- ✓ *12 cl of extra virgin olive oil*

1. *Preparation*
2. *Cut tomatoes into quarters. Then dip in boiling water, rinse with cold water and peel.*
3. *Put all the vegetables in a pan, salt and pepper. Add olive oil and place the lid on the pan.*
4. *Cook the vegetables over low heat for 45 minutes, stirring occasionally.*

Salad of roasted root vegetables

Ready in 25mins. 2 servings.

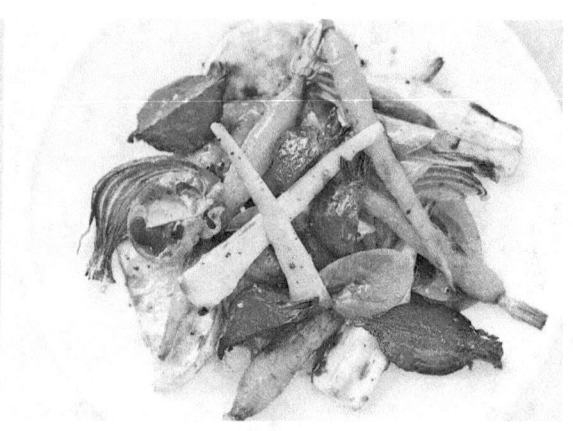

Ingredients
- ✓ 2 parsnips,
- ✓ 2 red beets,
- ✓ 1 sweet potato,
- ✓ 1 tablespoon olive oil
- ✓ 1 pinch dried oregano
- ✓ Salt and pepper
- ✓ Finely chopped fresh parsley (optional)

Preparation
1. Preheat oven to 200 degrees
2. Arrange the vegetables on a baking sheet in a single layer (make 2 batches if necessary).
3. Drizzle with olive oil, sprinkle with oregano, salt and pepper. Mix vegetables and roast in the oven for 15 to 20 minutes, until soft and golden.
4. Let cool and serve with feta cheese and fresh parsley.

Eastern lentil salad
Ready in 50 mins. 4 servings.

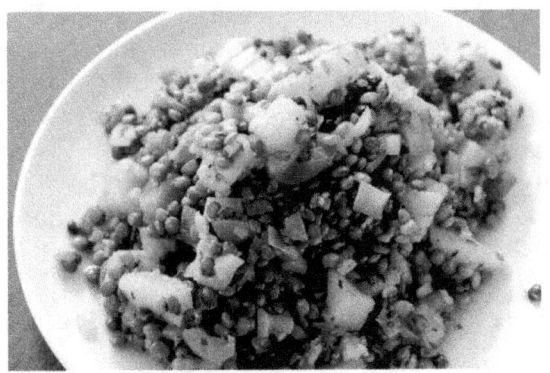

Ingredients
- ✓ *250 grams of lentils, green*
- ✓ *1 garlic clove*
- ✓ *1 good pinch of ground cumin*
- ✓ *1 untreated lemon slice*
- ✓ *1 small red onion, minced*
- ✓ *85 g of rehydrated dried apricots*
- ✓ *3 small peppers*
- ✓ *100 g broccoli florets halved*
- ✓ *50 g chopped dry goat cheese*
- ✓ *2 tbsp. tablespoons roasted sunflower seeds*
- ✓ *coriander*
- ✓ *juice of 1 lemon*
- ✓ *salt pepper*
- ✓ *3 tbsp. tablespoons of extra virgin olive oil*
- ✓ *2 tbsp. tablespoon chopped coriander*

Preparation
1. *Rinse lentils and place them in a large saucepan. Cover them well with cold water and bring to aboil.*
2. *Add the peeled garlic clove, cumin, and lemon slice. Reduce heat and simmer 25 to 40 minutes, depending on the variety of lenses: they are tender, without crashing.*
3. *Meanwhile, prepare the coriander. In a bowl, mix the lemon juice with salt and pepper until the salt is dissolved, then emulsify with the oil. Stir in the coriander.*
4. *Drain the lentils, remove garlic and lemon, and then pour in the bowl. Mix them with the coriander.*
5. *Add onion, apricots, peppers, and broccoli. Mix well. Sprinkle cheese and sunflower seeds. Serve.*

Greek salad

Ready in 35 mins. 4 servings.

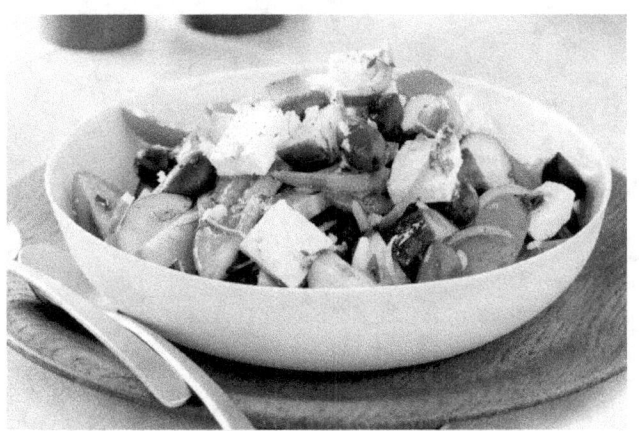

Ingredients
- ✓ *3 diced tomatoes*
- ✓ *1 green pepper, diced*
- ✓ *½ cucumber, diced*
- ✓ *1 small red onion, diced*
- ✓ *A handful of black olives*
- ✓ *75 g Feta*
- ✓ *3-4 tablespoons olive oil*
- ✓ *1 teaspoon red wine vinegar*
- ✓ *1 teaspoon lemon juice*
- ✓ *1 clove crushed garlic*
- ✓ *1/2 teaspoon dried oregano*
- ✓ *Salt and ground black pepper*

Preparation
1. *In a bowl, combine tomatoes, green pepper, onion, cucumber, and olives.*
2. *Prepare seasoning with oil, vinegar, lemon juice, garlic, oregano, salt, and pepper.*
3. *Pour over salad and let stand 30 minutes for well together flavors.*
4. *Add feta cheese and mix well before serving.*

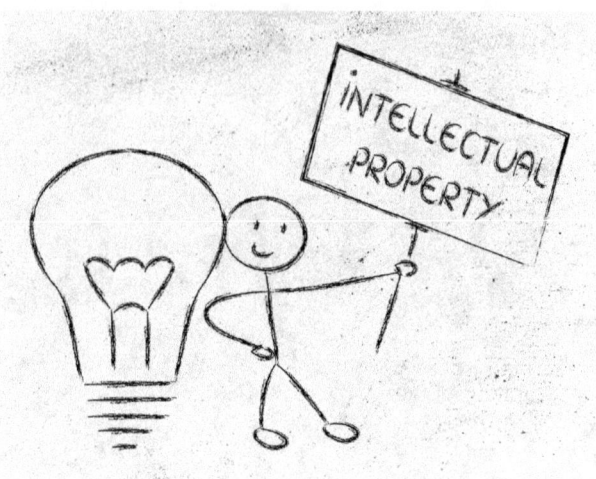

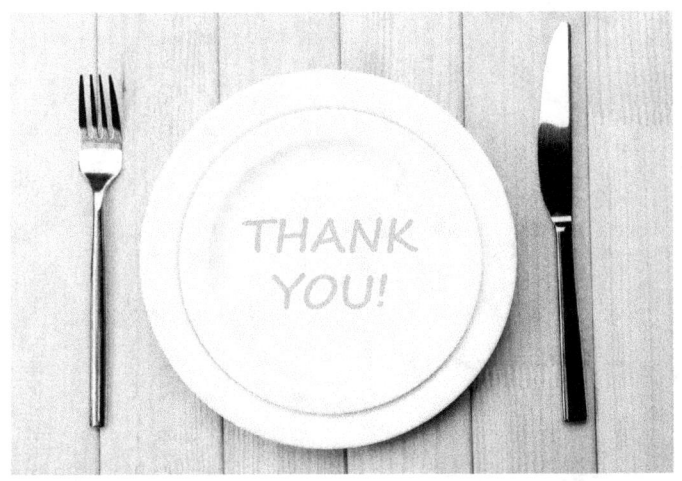

Thank you for purchasing ' Healthy Choice - 50 delicious creative vegetable salads' - We hope that it has shown you that cooking can be quick, simple and accessible to all. We also hope that it will inspire you with the desire to create more homemade meals and provide you with ideas to keep you and the kids fuelled by wholesome, plant-based food.